# ESSENTIAL OILS
## Therapeutic Bath
### *Soaking Recipes*

by Kathrine Townsend

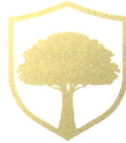

**CLADD**
PUBLISHING

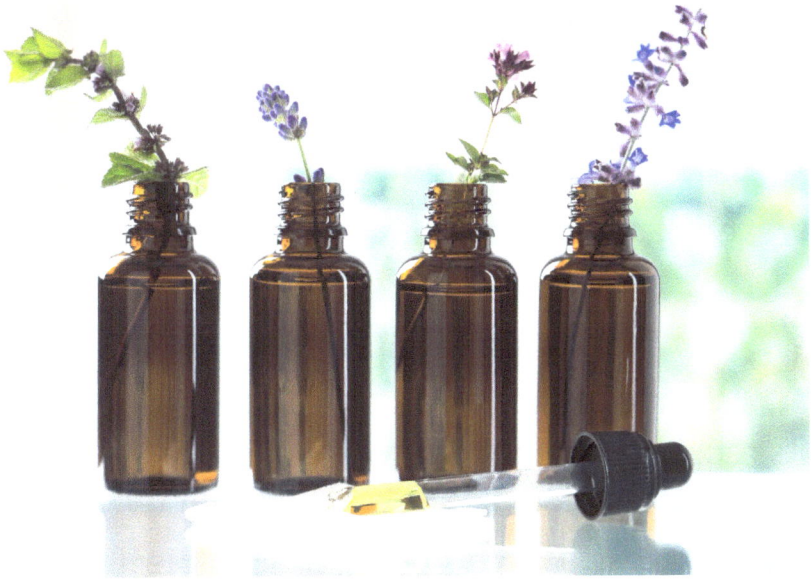

# Commonly Asked Questions

## Q: CAN I DO THESE RECIPES WITH LITTLE EXPERIENCE AND ON A BUDGET?

A: Yes, while the recipes are based on luxurious products they are budget friendly, non-toxic formulas. This is an excellent book for normal people wanting to enhance their life with high priced essential oil products; but do not want to purchase the expensive version from a specialty store.

## Q: WHAT DOES EO MEAN?

A: EO or EOs is the abbreviation for Essential Oils. It is commonly used and will be used in this book.

# Q: RAW, ORGANIC AND NATURAL

**A:** For the highest quality ingredients use raw and or cold pressed honey, coconut, shea butter, aloe vera, jojoba, beeswax, cocoa, and sweet almond oil. Try your best to obtain supplies that are organic and or natural.

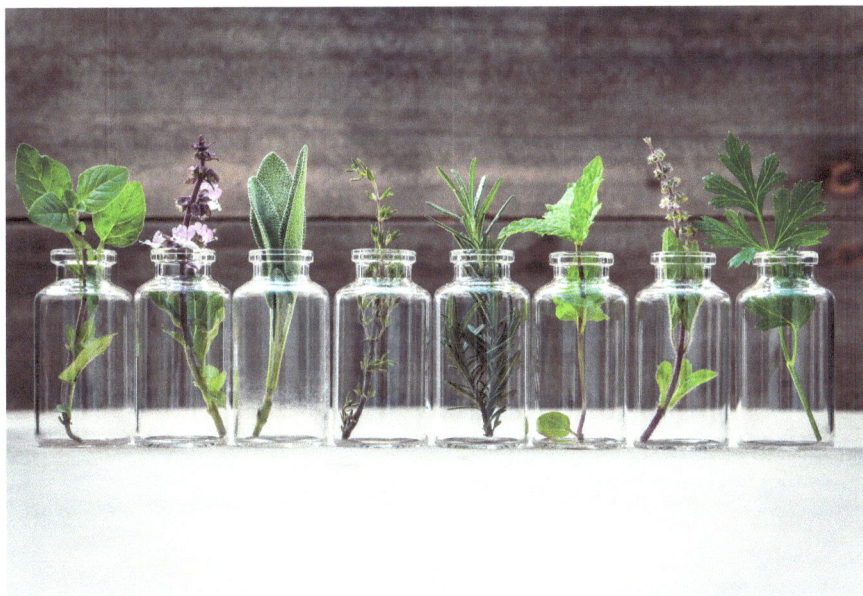

# Carrier Oils

The scent of EOs will evaporate quickly, unless combined with a carrier oil. Carrier oils usually come from the fatty portion of a plant and help the essential oils maintain their scent for long periods of time.

Carrier Oils are also important for diluting your EOs prior to ingesting or direct use on **the skin.**

# THESE ARE EXCELLENT CARRIER OILS:

- Almond Oil
- Jojoba Oil
- Olive Oil
- Grapeseed Oil
- Avocado Oil
- Coconut Oil

# 10 EOs to Avoid

Some EOs are not safe for skin contact or ingestion. They can cause skin problems or may even be poisonous.

## AVOID THESE ESSENTIAL OILS:

- Bitter Almond
- Calamus
- Horseradish
- Mugwort
- Mustard
- Rue
- Yellow Camphor
- Savin
- Southernwood
- Tansy

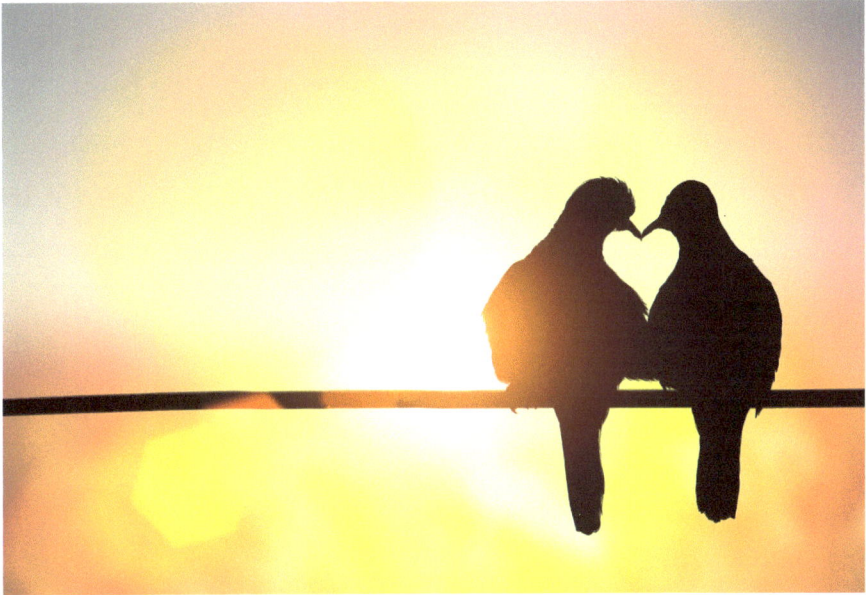

# Aphrodisiacs Oils

The following essential oils are excellent options to add to your baths soaks, for a sensual and relaxing aroma.

## YLANG YLANG

Ylang Ylang has a powerful floral aroma, and is an aphrodisiac. Has a feminine aroma.

## NEROLI

Neroli has a sweet floral aroma, which is very soothing to an overworked nervous system. Has a feminine aroma.

### Rose Absolute Bulgarian

This is a highly-prized EO and is one of the best aphrodisiacs. Rose has a deep floral aroma and is symbolic for the expression of love. *Has a feminine aroma.*

### Jasmine Absolute

Jasmine is an incredible aphrodisiac and sexual tonic. It is very calming to the mind and nervous system. It has deep, warm, floral notes. *Has a feminine aroma.*

### Sandalwood Australian

This has woody, balsamic, and earthy tones. Its aroma is valued for its ability to calm the mind. It is also used as a sexual tonic. *Has a masculine aroma.*

### Patchouli

It is well-known for its aphrodisiac properties. Patchouli is very grounding and intoxicating to the senses. Has a masculine aroma.

### Vetiver

This warm, smoky, woody EO is very relaxing. It gently sedates an overworked mind. Has a masculine aroma.

# Mix It Yourself Instructions

## 3 BASIC WAYS TO ADD ESSENTIAL OILS TO A BATH:

1. Add 5 drops of any EO to 1 Tbsp. of carrier oil, and then add to your bath water.
2. Add 5 drops of any EO to 1 cup of whole milk, then pour it into your bath.
3. Blend 5 drops of any EO into 2-oz. of bath salts and 2 teaspoon jojoba oil, then add to your bath.

## SKIN SOOTHING OILS:

- Lavender
- Roman Chamomile
- Vetiver
- Frankincense Myrrh

## BATH SALT CHEAT SHEET

Being able to mix your own bath salts is something every person should know. Bath salts provide detoxification of your entire body. When the essential oils are added to the salt, in addition to the heat of the water, you will experience a total mind and body purge.

## BASE RECIPE

- 1 cup Epsom salt
- 1 cup kosher salt
- ½ cup baking soda
- 12- 20 drops any essential oil or combination

## Instructions:

1. Combine salts and baking soda in a jar
2. Stir in desired essential oils
3. Store in cool, dark place
4. Use about ¼ cup per bath

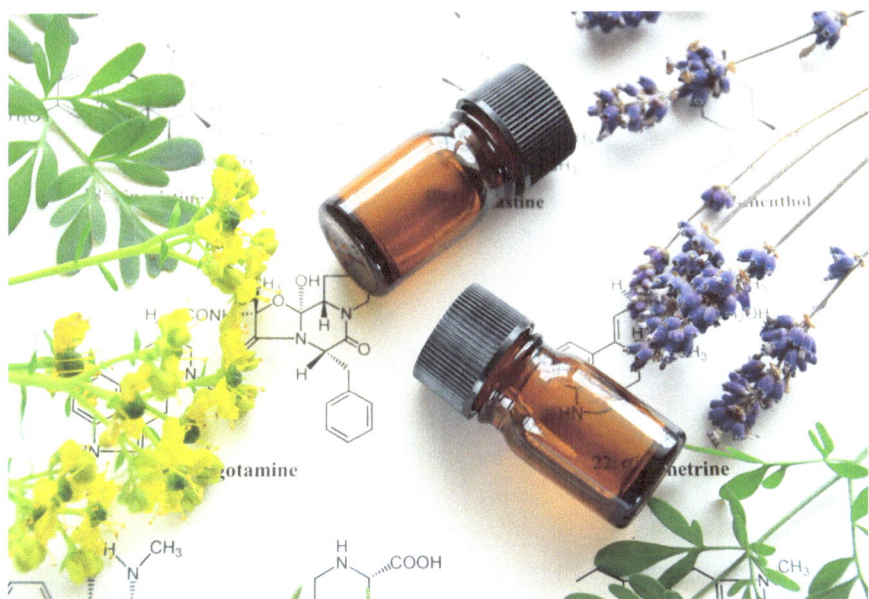

# Essential Oil Combinations

## SINUS RELIEF
8 drops eucalyptus + 8 drops peppermint

## PHYSICAL RELAXATION
9 drops lavender + 10 drops bergamot

## MENTAL RELAXATION
8 drops lemon + 8 drops rosemary

## RELEASE
8 drops sage + 3 drops mint + 4 drops tea tree

## SOOTHING

4 drops geranium + 9 drops lavender + 5 drops rose

## UPLIFTING

5 drops orange + 4 drops clove + 4 drops cedarwood + 5 drops lemon

# Detoxing Combinations

ADD 3-4 DROPS OF EACH ESSENTIAL OIL COMBINATION TO THE SALT AND BAKING SODA MIXTURE.

- Peppermint, tangerine, grapefruit
- Copaiba, wintergreen, panaway
- Lavender, lemon, peppermint
- Helichrysum, lavender, melrose
- Peppermint, chamomile, and Copaiba
- Idaho blue spruce, Ylang Ylang

## BATH SALT BENEFITS

- Stress relief
- Reducing muscle aches
- Improving circulation
- Better nutrient absorption
- Headache relief
- Speeding up wound healing
- During illness, especially respiratory illness
- For children to help mineral absorption and improve sleep
- For acne, eczema or other skin problems
- For joint pain relief

- To help relieve poison ivy or skin reactions
- Improving skin hydration

## BAKING SODA BENEFITS

Your body loves sodium bicarbonate. Bicarbonate ions occur naturally in our bloodstream to aid in maintaining our acid/alkaline balance. It transports carbon dioxide from our tissues, to the lungs to be expelled. Sodium bicarbonate is also found in our saliva as an acid reducer.

The medicinal benefits go beyond comprehension; as renowned cancer and disease experts are now showing the lifesaving benefits of baking soda.

## AILMENTS ITS KNOWN TO TREAT:

- Anti-fungal
- It is a natural, potent and non-toxic medicine
- High quality therapeutic agent
- Body and skin cleanser and care
- Increases your body's natural pH (alkalinity) levels
- Deodorizer
- And many more

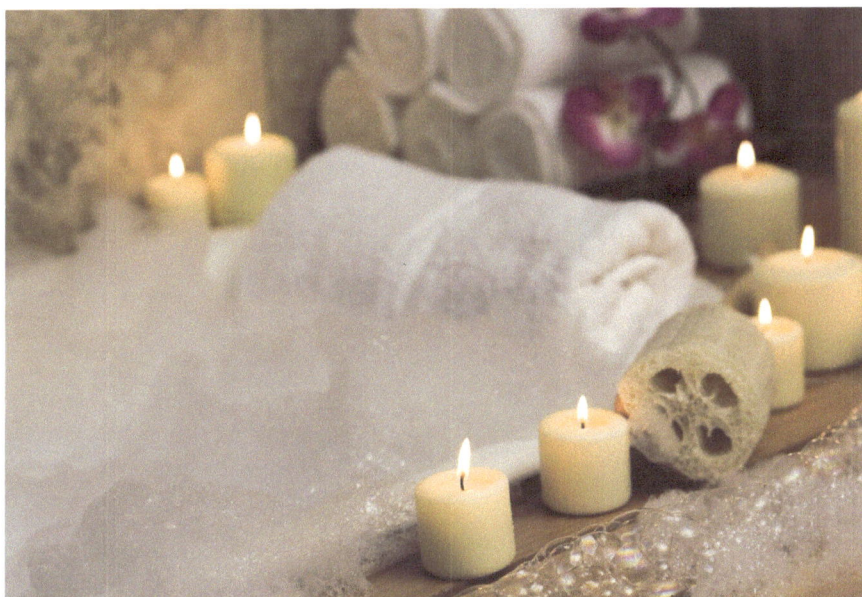

# Chicken Pox – Hives – Measles

If you are suffering from chicken pox, hives, or measles then try this bath soak. It will reduce the severe itchiness and stimulates healing.

## How To:
- Run a warm bath
- Put in ½ cup of baking soda
- 5 drops Chamomile EO
- 5 drops Jasmine EO
- Soak in the tub until water cools
- Towel off when done

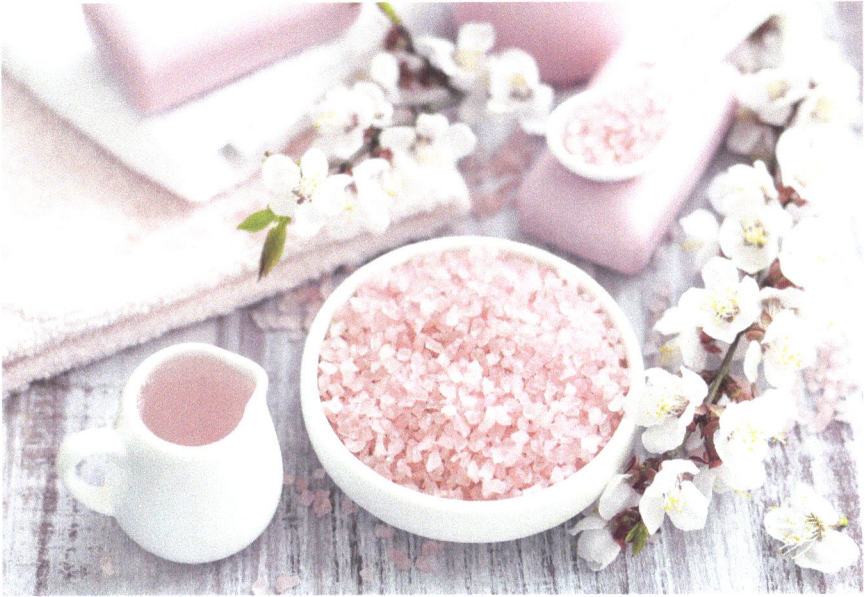

# Detox Serenity

This is an incredible detoxing bath therapy, used to remove heavy metals, toxins, chemicals, medication residue, exposure to radiation, and unclogs pores.

## Ingredients:
- 1 cup Himalayan pink salt
- 1 cup dead sea salt
- 1 cup Epsom salt
- 5 tsp fractionated coconut oil
- 13 drops of clary sage EO
- 13 drops of lemongrass EO

## How To:

- Use 1 large ball mason jar
- add all salts together
- Mix in fractionated coconut oil
- Clary sage EO
- Lemongrass EO
- Add ¼ of the bath salts to running bath water.
- Mix well and allow the salt grains to dissolve
- Soak for 25 to 30 minutes
- Quickly rinse off and pat dry (optional)

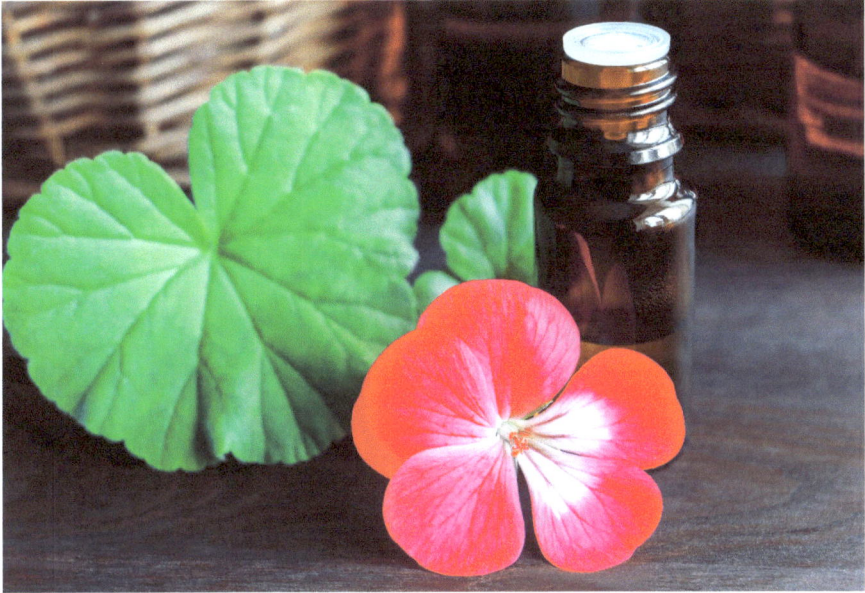

# Harmony & Appreciation

The essential oils combination balances your mind, body and spirit. Close your eyes and reminisce on all the wonderful things in your life. When you are finished you will feel in harmony with nature.

## How To:
- Combine 4 tablespoons of jojoba oil
- 12 drops geranium EO
- 6 drops sandalwood EO
- 6 drops lemon EO
- 2 drops clary sage EO
- Add to a warm bath and soak

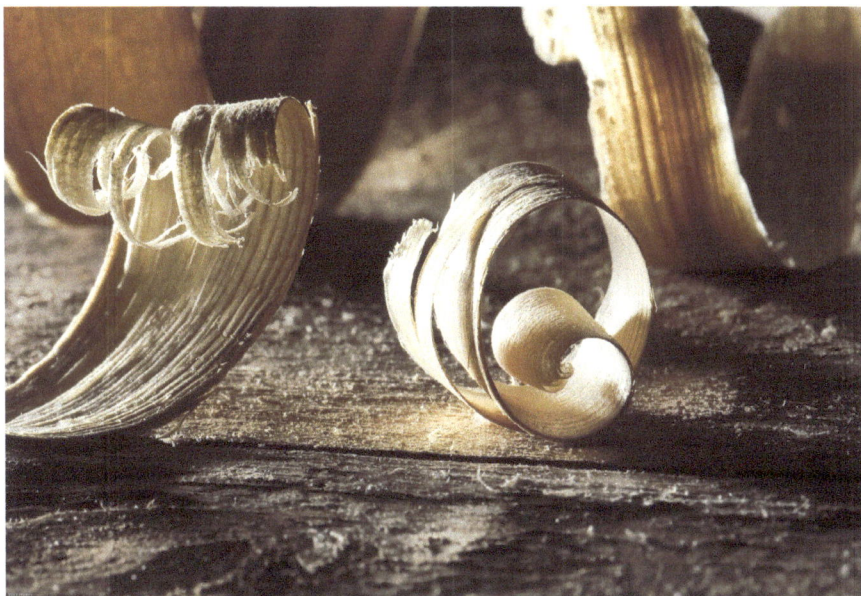

# The Good Life Mood Enhancer

## How To:

- Combine 4 tablespoons of jojoba oil
- 12 drops sandalwood EO
- 8 drops orange EO
- 4 drops rose EO
- 2 drops pine EO
- 2 drops lemon EO
- Add to a warm bath and soak

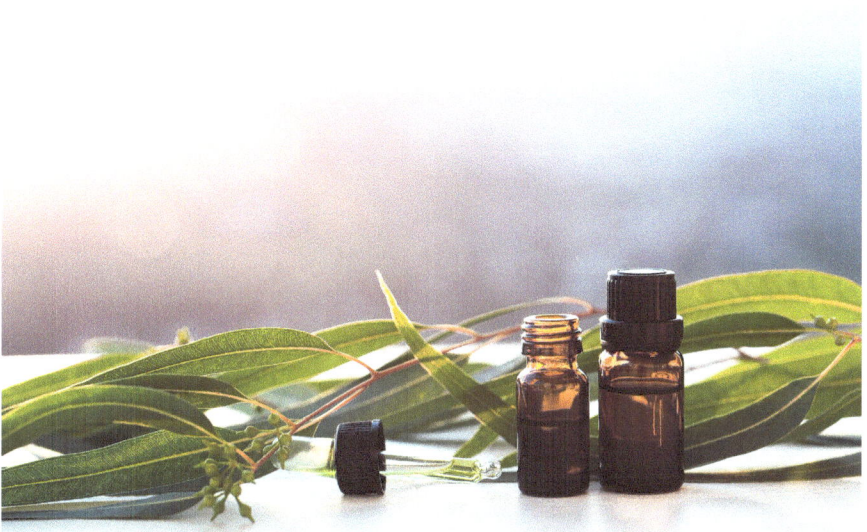

# Positive Uplifting Attitude

## How To:

- Mix 13 drops eucalyptus EO
- 8 drops lemon EO
- 4-5 drops cedarwood EO
- 4 oz. of grapeseed EO
- In glass jar
- Add 1 Tbsp. of mixture to a warm bath

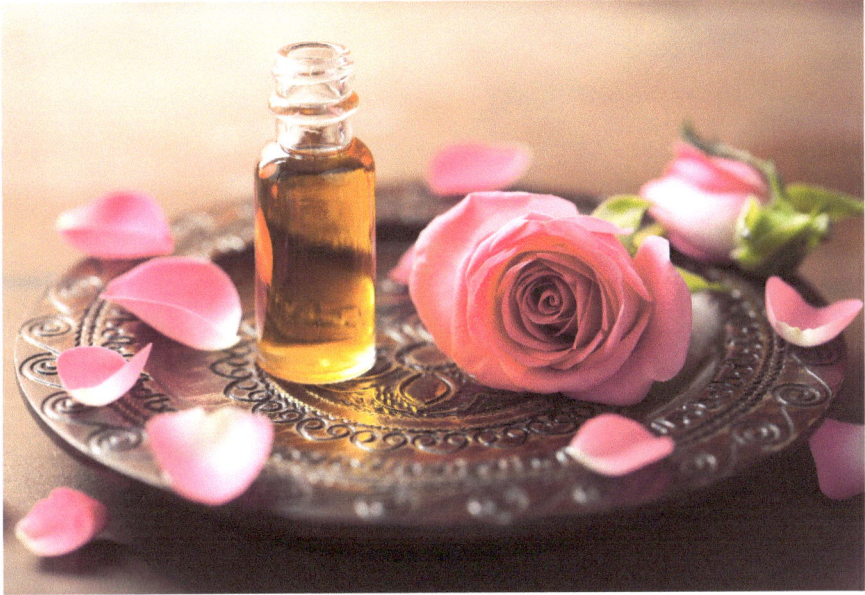

# Summer Morning Glory

This is a glorious morning bath soak. Start off your day with the enchanting aroma of these beautiful floral essential oils.

## How To:

- Combine 4 tablespoons of jojoba oil
- 10 drops sandalwood EO
- 5 drops jasmine EO
- 5 drops rose EO
- 5 drops bergamot EO
- Add to your warm bath

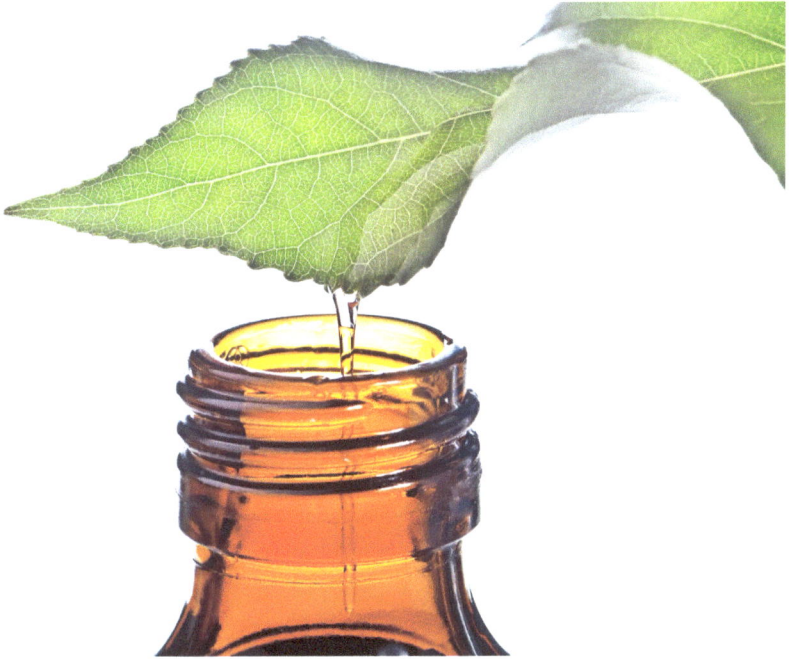

# Fungal Foot Soak

## Ingredients:

- Combine 5 drops of tea tree EO
- 1 drop of lemon EO
- 1 tablespoon of baking soda
- 1 tablespoon of Epsom salt
- 2 tablespoons of cider vinegar
- Add to your warm bath

# How To:

- Mix all the ingredients in a bowl of warm water
- Soak your feet for 5-15 minutes
- Dry your feet with a clean cloth

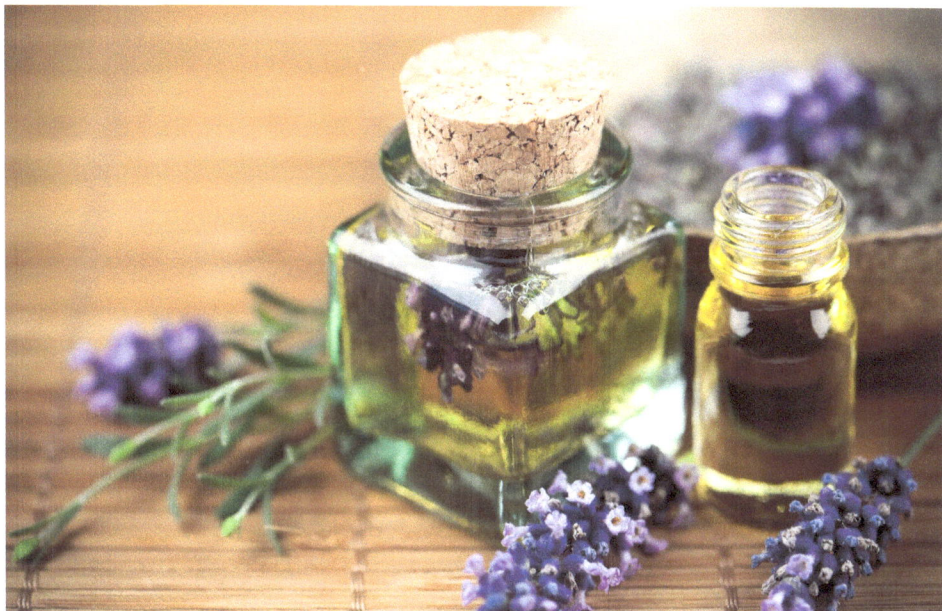

# Intense Moisture Therapy

## Ingredients:

- 2 ounces jojoba oil
- 8 drops lavender EO
- 8 drops geranium EO

## How To:

- In an amber glass bottle
- Mix all ingredients together
- Add 5 ml to your warm bath water, stir well and have a long soak

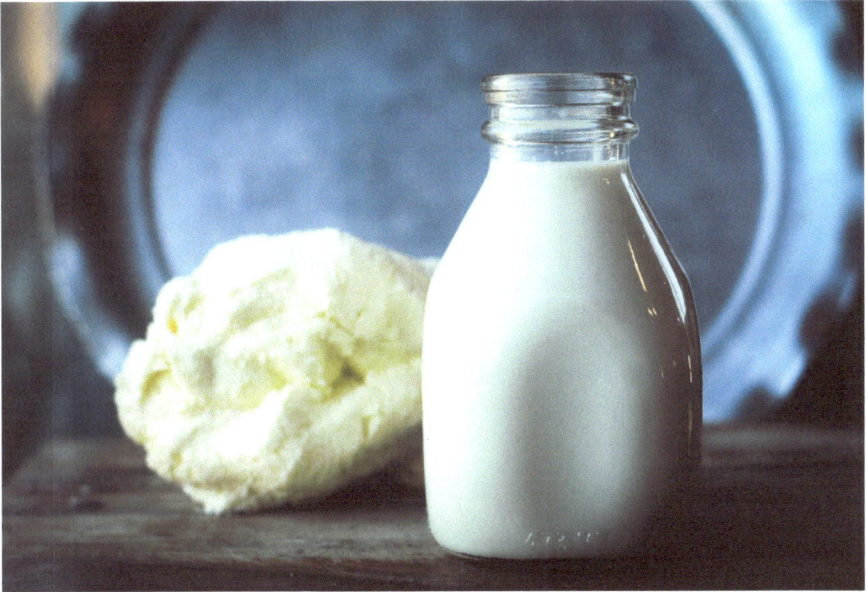

# Melt Your Stress Away

## How To:

- Add 5 drops of chamomile EO
- With 2 Tbsp. of whole milk
- Add to a warm bath and soak

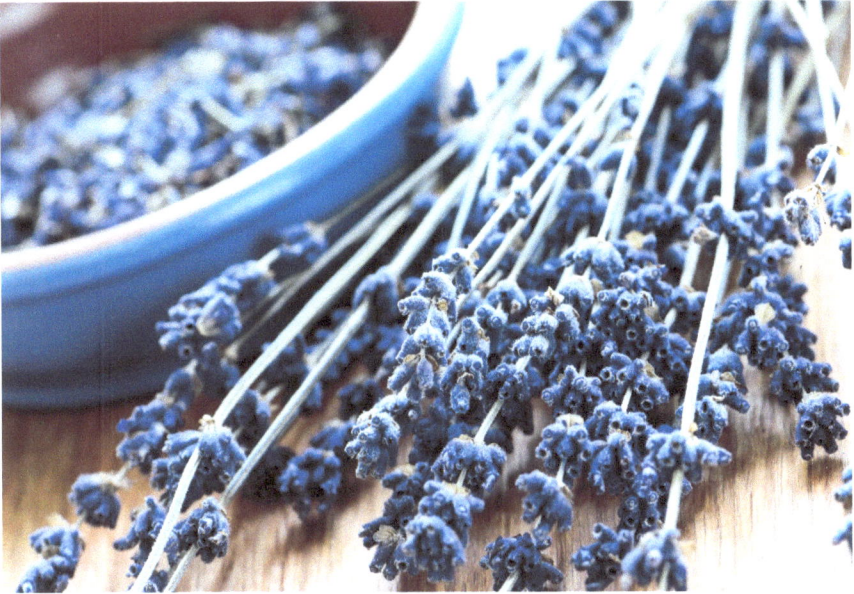

# Lavender Heaven

## How To:

- 2 cups Epsom Salts
- 1/2 cup dry lavender
- 5-6 drops pure lavender EO
- 10 drops pure eucalyptus EO
- Combine all ingredients in a small bowl
- fill bathtub with very warm water
- Use half or all the mixture
- soak for about 20 to 30 minutes

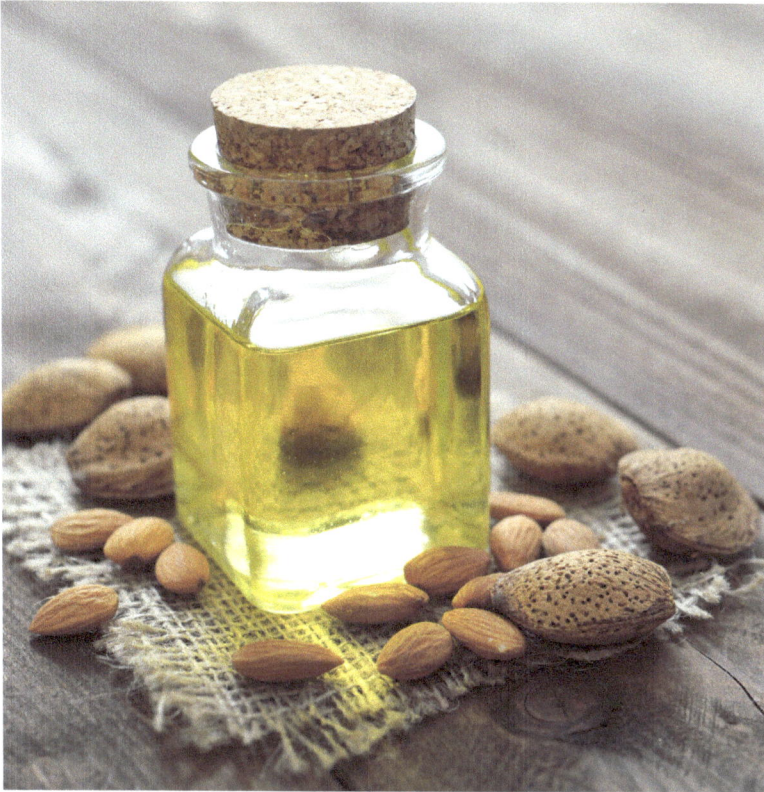

# Soothing Sunset

Soothing sunset is the best remedy for reducing entire body inflammation, relieve aches and pains, muscle cramps, muscle relaxer, remove toxins, a natural emollient for your skin, and reduces lactic acid build-up. Feel the magic of body and mind!

**Ingredients:**
- 3 cups Epsom salts
- 1 Tbsp. sweet almond oil

- 3 drops lemongrass EO
- 3 drops basil EO
- 3 drops lavender EO
- 2 drops lime EO
- 6 drops wintergreen EO
- 6 drops rosemary EO
- 6 drops peppermint EO
- 4 drops bergamot EO
- 4 drops douglas fir EO
- 4 drops ginger EO
- 2 drops marjoram EO
- 5 drops lavender EO
- 4 drops rosemary EO

## How To:

- Put the Epsom salts into a quart sized mason jar
- Drip the essential oils onto the salts and add the carrier oil
- Close tightly and shake well
- Use ¼ cup in a warm bath
- Soak for at least 20 minutes to relieve soreness from overworked muscles

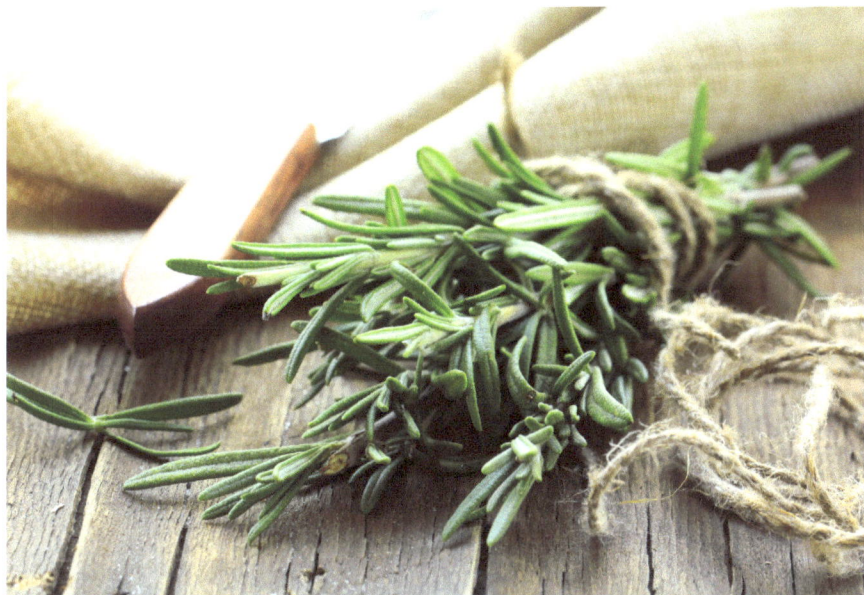

# Rosemary Renaissance

Soak in this Eucalyptus bath for purifying, oxygenating, energizing and detoxifying effects. Works wonders for general sore muscles, feet, upper and lower back pain.

## Ingredients:
- 1 Cup Epsom Salts
- 1/4 Cup Sea Salts
- 1/4 Cup Baking Soda
- 3 drops each of Eucalyptus EO
- 3 drops Rosemary EO

# How To:

- Mix all ingredients together in a small bowl
- Begin filling bathtub with hot water
- Place the mixture under the faucet as it is filling
- Soak for at least 20 minutes
- Do a quick rinse
- Pat dry with a towel
- Go bed immediately as you may become very drowsy

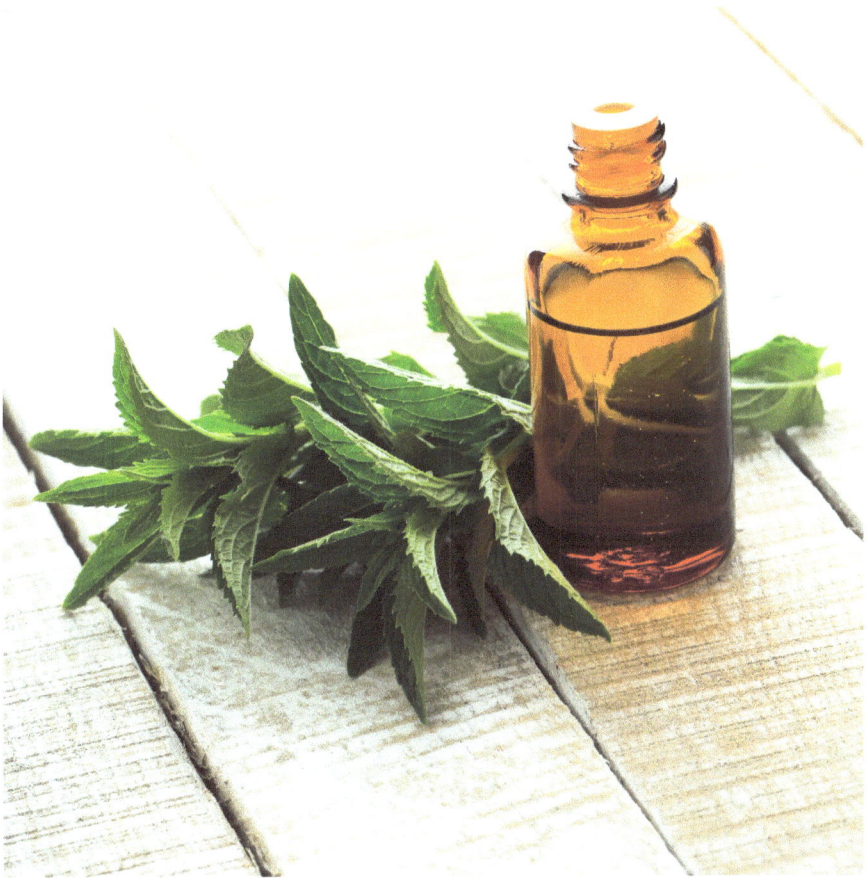

# Peppermint Sport Soak

Refreshing salt soak for sore muscles caused by a heavy workout.

## Ingredients:

- 5 drops lavender EO
- 2 drops peppermint EO
- 2 drops citrus EO
- 1 drops clove EO

- 1 Tbsp. jojoba oil

## How To:
- Fill your bathtub
- Mix all EOs in jojoba oil
- Pour into a warm bath
- Soak for at least 20 minutes
- Do a quick rinse
- Pat dry with a towel
- Go bed immediately as you may become very drowsy

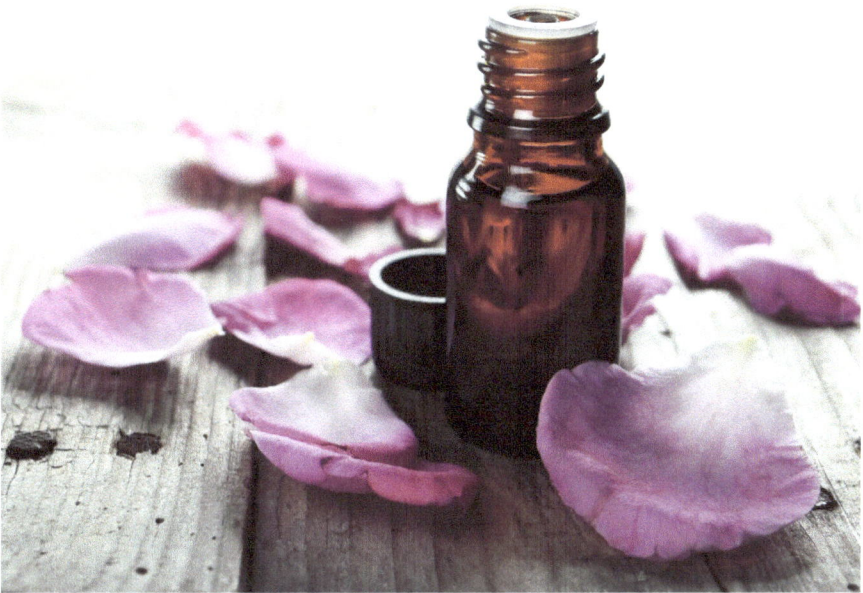

# Soothed Nerves

## How To:

- Add 16 drops lavender EO
- 9 drops geranium EO
- 4 drops lemongrass EO
- 4 oz. jojoba oil
- Store in a glass jar
- Add 1 Tbsp. of the mixture into a warm bath

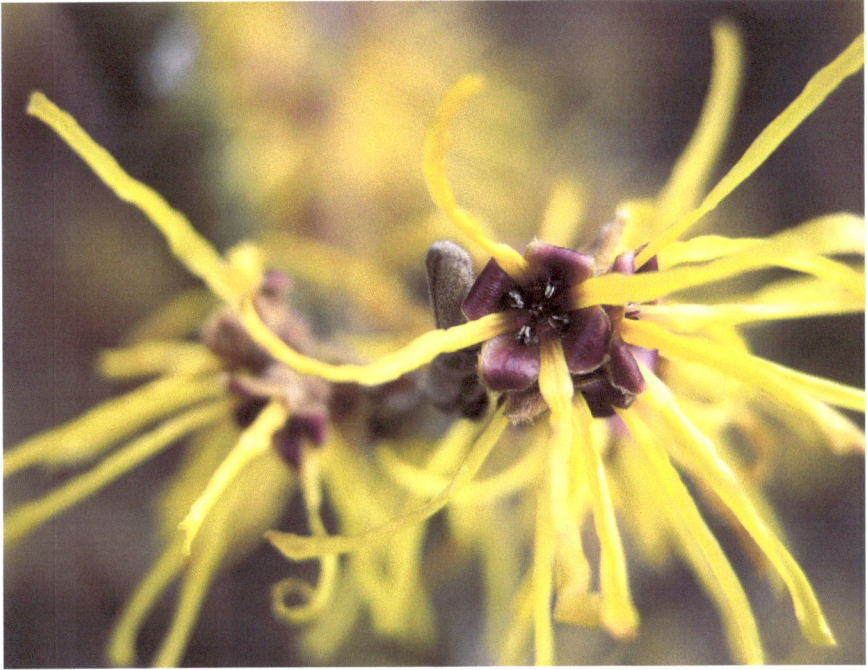

# Lights Out

## How To:

- Add 18 drops lavender EO
- 7 drops sandalwood EO
- 4 drops vetiver EO
- 2 drops ylang ylang EO
- 4 oz. sweet almond oil
- Combine all ingredients into a glass jar
- Add 1 Tbsp. of mixture into a warm bath

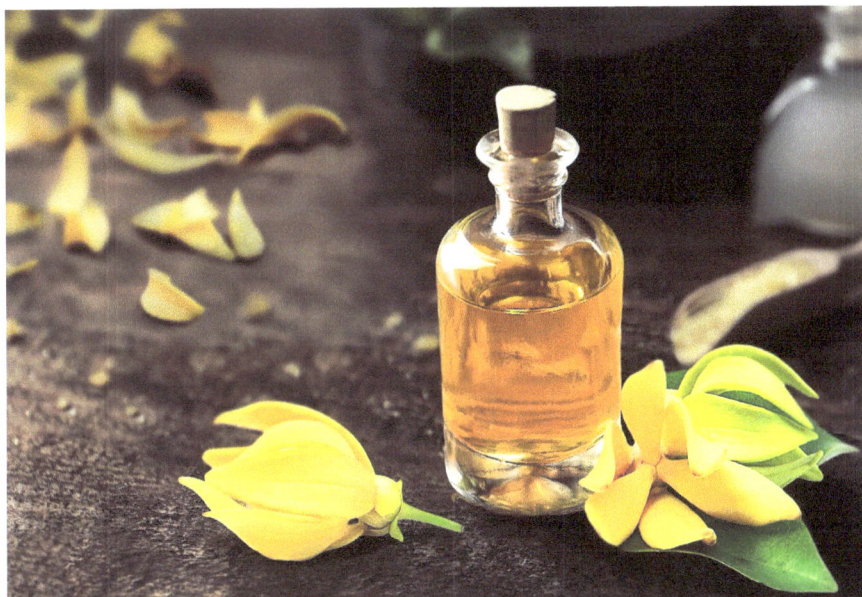

# Tension Headache Relief

This is a great way to release tension from your back, shoulders and neck area. The EO combination is excellent after a long day at work, or right before bed.

## How To:
- 2 drops Lavender EO
- 3 drops Chamomile EO
- 3 drops Rose EO
- Run a warm bath, add all ingredients and soak.

www.ingramcontent.com/pod-product-compliance
Lightning Source LLC
LaVergne TN
LVHW010023070426
835508LV00001B/24